THE EA

LEAN AND GREEN

FOR YOUR FIRST COURSES AND SOUP

50 step-by-step easy recipes for a Lean and Green food for your first courses and soup to burn fat fast and boost energy

Josephine Reed

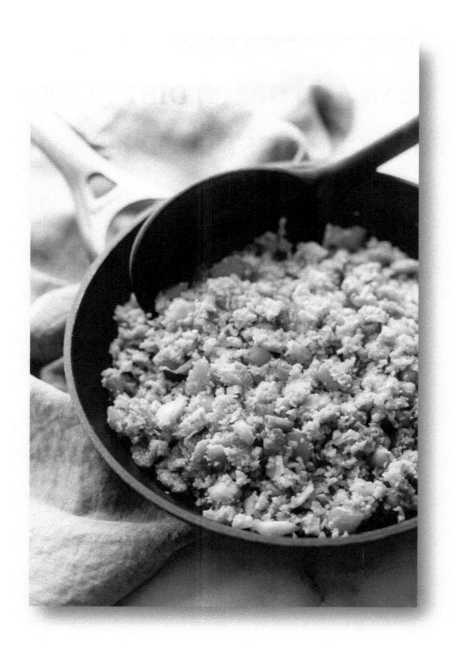

Table of contents

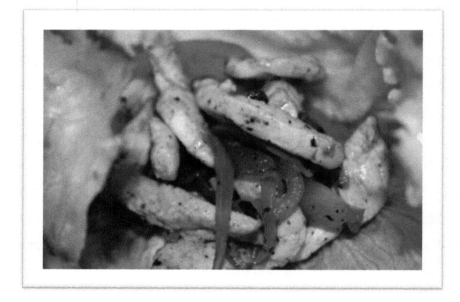

Coconut Battered Cauliflower Bites

Prep Time: 5 minutes

Cook Time: 20 minutes

Serve: 1

Ingredients:

- Salt and pepper to taste
- 1 flax egg or one tablespoon flaxseed meal + 3 tablespoon water
- 1 small cauliflower, cut into florets
- 1 teaspoon mixed spice
- ½ teaspoon mustard powder
- 2 tablespoons maple syrup
- 1 clove of garlic, minced
- 2 tablespoons soy sauce
- 1/3 cup oats flour
- 1/3 cup plain flour
- 1/3 cup desiccated coconut

Instructions:

1. Prepare the ingredients.

2. In a mixing bowl, mix oats, flour, and desiccated coconut. Season with salt and pepper to taste. Set aside.

3. In another bowl, place the flax egg and add a pinch of salt to taste. Set aside.

4. Season the cauliflower with mixed spice and mustard powder.

5. Dredge the florets in the flax egg first, then in the flour mixture.

6. Air Frying. Place inside the Instant Crisp Air Fryer, lock the air fryer lid and cook at 400°F or 15 minutes.

7. Meanwhile, place the maple syrup, garlic, and soy sauce in a saucepan and heat over medium flame. Wait for it to boil and adjust the heat to low until the sauce thickens.

8. After 15 minutes, take out the florets from the Instant Crisp Air Fryer and place them in the saucepan.

9. Toss to coat the florets and place inside the Instant Crisp Air Fryer and cook for another 5 minutes.

Nutrition: Calories: 154, Fat: 2.3g, Protein: 4.69g

Crispy Jalapeno Coins

Prep Time: 10 minutes

Cook Time: 5 minutes

Serve: 1

Ingredients:

- 1 egg
- 2–3 tablespoon coconut flour
- 1 sliced and seeded jalapeno
- Pinch garlic powder
- Pinch onion powder
- Bit cajun seasoning (optional)
- Pinch pepper and salt

Instructions:

1. Prepare the ingredients. Ensure your Instant Crisp Air Fryer is preheated to 400 degrees.

2. Mix all dry ingredients.

3. Pat jalapeno slices dry. Dip coins into the egg wash and then into the dry mixture. Toss to coat thoroughly.

4. Add coated jalapeno slices to Instant Crisp Air Fryer in a singular layer. Spray with olive oil.

5. Air Frying. Lock the air fryer lid. Set temperature to 350°F and set time to 5 minutes. Cook just till crispy.

Nutrition: Calories: 128, Fat: 8g, Protein: 7g, Sugar: 0g

Buffalo Cauliflower

Prep Time: 5 minutes

Cook Time: 15 minutes

Serve: 1

Ingredients:

Cauliflower

- 1 cup panko breadcrumbs
- 1 teaspoon salt
- 2 cup cauliflower florets

Buffalo Coating

- ¼ cup vegan buffalo sauce
- ¼ cup melted vegan butter

Instructions:

1. Prepare the ingredients. Melt butter in microwave and whisk in buffalo sauce.

2. Dip each cauliflower floret into a buffalo mixture, ensuring it gets coated well. Holdover a bowl till the floret is done dripping.

3. Mix breadcrumbs with salt.

4. Air Frying. Dredge dipped florets into breadcrumbs and place them into Instant Crisp Air Fryer. Lock the air fryer lid. Set

temperature to 350°F and set time to 15 minutes. When slightly browned, they are ready to eat!

5. Serve with your favorite Keto dipping sauce!

Nutrition: Calories: 194, Fat: 17g, Protein: 10g, Sugar: 3

Cream of Cauliflower

Prep Time: 1 hour

Cook Time: 1 hour

Serve: 4

Ingredients:

- Salt and pepper
- ½ cup (120 ml) heavy cream
- ½ teaspoon guar or xanthan (optional)
- 1 package or 285 g frozen cauliflower
- 1 quart (960 ml) chicken broth
- ¾ cup (90 g) diced celery
- ¾ cup (120 g) diced onion
- tablespoons (42 g) butter

Instructions:

1. Melt the buutter and sauté the onion and celery in it until they are floppy. Incorporate this in a large saucepan with the cauliflower and chicken broth and cook until the cauliflower is soft.

2.Using a slotted spoon to pass the vegetables to a blender, and add in the broth as much as you want. Add (if using) guar or xanthan and purée the ingredients.

3.Pour back the paste into the saucepan. Add salt and some pepper into the mix with some cream.

Nutrition: 9,5 g. carbo. and 3 g. fiber, for a total of 6,5 grams of usable carbs and 7 grams of protein.

California Soup

Prep Time: 10 min

Cook Time: 10 min

Serve: 3

Ingredients:

- 1 quart (960 ml) chicken broth, heated
- 1 large or 2 small, very ripe black avocados, pitted, peeled, and cut into chunks

Instructions:

1.Add the avocados with the broth in a blender puree until very smooth and serve.

Nutrition: 3,5 g. carbo. and 1,5 g. fiber, total of 2,5 grams of usable carbs and 4 grams of protein.

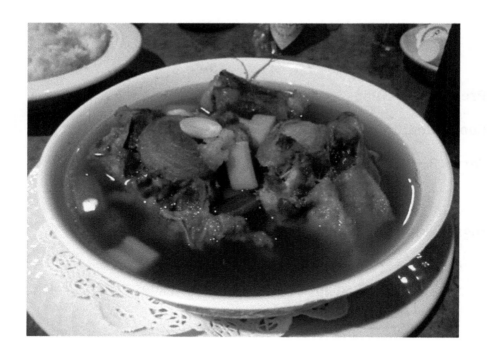

Cheesy Cauliflower Soup

Prep Time: 15 min

Cook Time: 1 hour

Serve: 5

Ingredients:

- 1 tablespoon (6 g) minced scallion
- slices bacon, cooked and drained
- Guar or xanthan (optional)
- 1½ cups (180 g) shredded cheddar cheese
- 1½ cups (360 ml) Carb Countdown dairy beverage or half-and-half
- teaspoons white vinegar
- 1 teaspoon salt
- cups (720 ml) chicken broth
- 1 tablespoon (7 g) grated carrot
- 2 tablespoons (20 g) finely chopped celery
- 1 tablespoon (10 g) finely chopped onion
- cups (600 g) cauliflower, diced small

Instructions:

1.In a big, heavy-bottomed pan, placed the cauliflower, onion, celery, and carrot. Add the broth, salt, and vinegar to the chicken; bring it to a simmer and cook for about 30 to 45 minutes.

2.Stir in the Carb Countdown or half-and-half and then whisk in the cheese a bit at a time before adding more, allowing each additional time to melt. With guar or xanthan, thicken it a bit if you think it needs it.

3.Cover each serving with slightly crumbled bacon and hazelnuts.

Nutrition: 17 g protein; 7 g carbohydrate; 2 g dietary fiber; 5 g usable carbs.

Egg drop Soup

Prep Time: 10 min

Cook Time: 10 min

Serve: 3

Ingredients:

- eggs
- 1 scallion, sliced
- ½ teaspoon grated fresh ginger
- 1 tablespoon (15 ml) rice vinegar
- 1 tablespoon (15 ml) soy sauce
- ¼ teaspoon guar (optional)
- 1 quart (960 ml) chicken broth

Instructions:

1.Put 1 cup (240 ml) or so of the chicken stock in your processor, turn it on medium, and add the guar (if using). Let it mix for a moment, and then put it in a big saucepan with the broth's rest. (If you're not using the guar, then put all the liquid directly in a saucepan.)

2.Put in the rice vinegar, soy sauce, ginger, and scallion. Heat over medium-high heat and let it boil for 5-10 minutes to let the flavors mix.

3.Beat the eggs in a glass mixing cup or small pitcher — something with a pouring edge. Using a fork to stir the soup's surface in a gradual circle and pour in about ¼ of the eggs, stirring while cooking and turning into shreds (which can occur almost instantly). Do three more times, using up half the egg.

Nutrition: 2 g. carbo. | a trace of fiber, and 8 grams of protein.

Cauliflower, Spinach, and Cheese Soup

Prep Time: 6 hours

Cook Time: 1 1/2 hour

Serve: 8

Ingredients:

- 1 cup (240 ml) Carb Countdown dairy beverage
- Gouda cheese
- cups (675 g) shredded smoked
- cloves garlic, crushed
- ¼ teaspoon pepper
- ½ teaspoon salt or Vega-Sal
- ¼ teaspoon cayenne
- ounces (140 g) bagged baby spinach leaves, pre-washed
- ½ cup (80 g) minced red onion
- 1 quart (960 ml) chicken broth
- Guar or xanthan
- cups (900 g) cauliflower florets, cut into ½-inch (1.3-cm) pieces

Instructions:

1.Combine the broth, cauliflower, onion, spinach, cayenne, or Vega-Sal salt, pepper, and garlic in your slow cooker. Close the slow cooker, set it to low, and let simmer for 6 hours or until tender.

2.Stir in the Gouda when the time's up, a little at a time, and then the Carb Timer. Cover the slow cooker again and steam for another 15 minutes or until the cheese has melted completely. Slightly thicken the broth with guar or xanthan.

Nutrition: 17 g protein, 7 g carbohydrate, 2 g dietary fiber, 5 g usable carbs.

Corner-Filling Soup

Prep Time: 1/2 hour

Cook Time: 1/2 hour

Serve: 6

Ingredients:

- ¼ teaspoon pepper
- tablespoons (30 ml) dry sherry
- 1 quart (960 ml) beef broth
- 1 small onion, sliced paper-thin
- ounces (115 g) sliced mushrooms
- 2 tablespoons (28 g) butter

Instructions:

1. In a pot, heat the butter and sauté the mushrooms and onions into the butter until they're soft.

2. Apply the broth, sherry, and pepper over the meat. For 5-10 minutes or so, let it steam, just to change the flavors a bit, and serve.

Nutrition: 5,5 grams of carbohydrates and 1,1 gram of fiber, for a total of 4,5 grams of usable carbs and 8 grams of protein.

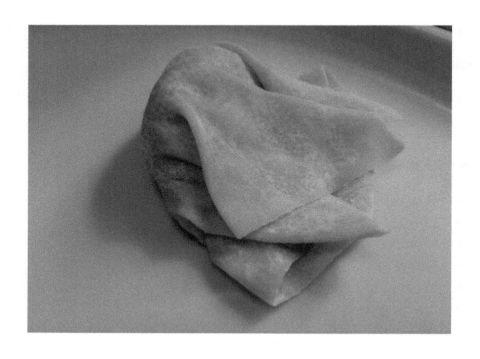

Stracciatella

Prep Time: 15 min

Cook Time: 45 min

Serve: 4-6

Ingredients:

- ½ teaspoon dried marjoram
- Pinch of nutmeg
- ½ teaspoon lemon juice
- ½ cup (50 g) grated Parmesan cheese
- eggs
- 1 quart (960 ml) chicken broth, divided

Instructions:

1.In a glass measuring cup or large pitcher, place 1/4 cup (60 ml) of the broth. Over medium heat, spill the remainder into a large saucepan.

2.In a measuring cup, add the eggs to the broth and beat them with a fork. Apply the lemon juice, Parmesan, and nutmeg, and then beat until well mixed using a fork.

3.Stir it using a fork as you add small quantities of the egg and cheese mixture until it is all mixed in while the broth in the saucepan is boiling. (Don't allow this to create long scraps like

Chinese egg drop soup; instead, it makes small, fluffy particles because of the Parmesan.)

4.Apply the marjoram, smash it between your fingers a little bit, and steam the soup for a minute or two before serving.

Nutrition: 2 grams of carbohydrates, a trace of fiber, and 12 grams of protein.

Peanut Soup

Prep Time: 15 min

Cook Time: 45 min

Serve: 5-7

Ingredients:

- Salted peanuts, chopped
- cups (420 ml) half-and-half or heavy cream
- 1 teaspoon guar gum (optional)
- 1¼ cups (325 g) natural peanut butter (Here, we used smooth.)
- ½ teaspoon salt or Vega-Sal
- quarts (1.9 L) chicken broth
- 1 medium onion, finely chopped
- 2 or 3 ribs celery, finely chopped
- tablespoons (42 g) butter

Instruction:

1.Melt the butter in a pot, then sauté the butter with the celery and onion.

2.Stir in the broth, salt, and peanut butter.

3.Cover and cook for at least 60 minutes at the lowest temperature, stirring now and then.

4.If you are using guar gum (without adding carbohydrates, it makes the soup thicker; scoop 1 cup (245 ml) of the soup out of the pot about 16 minutes before serving.

5.to this cup, apply the guar gum, run the mixture for a couple of seconds through the blender and whisk it back into the broth.

6.Stir in half-and-a-half and cook for 15 minutes more. Connect the peanuts to the garnish.

Nutrition: 19 grams of carbohydrates and 3 grams of fiber in each serving, with 16 grams of available carbohydrates and 29 grams of protein.

Soap De Frijoles Negros

Prep Time: 15 min

Cook Time: 45 min

Serve: 6-8

Ingredients:

- ¼ cup (16 g) chopped cilantro
- ½ cup (115 g) plain yogurt
- ½ teaspoon salt or Vega-Sal
- ½ teaspoon red pepper flakes
- 1 tablespoon (6.3 g) ground cumin
- tablespoons (30 ml) lime juice
- 1 cup (130 g) salsa
- cloves garlic, crushed
- ½ cup (80 g) chopped onion
- 1 tablespoon (15 ml) olive oil
- 1 can (14½ ounces, or 411 ml) chicken broth
- 1 can (15 ounces, or 420 g) black beans
- 2 cans (15 ounces, or 420 g) Eden brand black soybeans

Instructions:

1.With the S-blade in place, bring half of the beans and half of the chicken broth into your blender or in your food processor. Run the unit before it purées the beans. Transfer the mixture and purée the other half of the beans and the other half of the chicken broth into a bowl that contains at least 2 quarts (1.9 L). To the first batch, add it.

2.Heat the olive oil over medium-low-heat in a heavy-bottomed saucepan and put in the onion. Sauté until the onion becomes transparent. Add the garlic and bean purée. Now incorporate sauce, lime juice, cumin, flakes of red pepper, and salt or Vega-Sal. Once the soup is cooked through, turn the heat up a little and then turn it back down to the lowest level and let it boil for 30 to 45 minutes. Serve with a dollop of plain-yogurt and a sprinkle of minced cilantro (or sour cream, if you prefer).

Nutrition: 18 g of protein, 25 g of fiber, 13 g of dietary fiber, 13 g of available carbohydrates.

Artichoke Soup

Prep Time: 15 min

Cook Time: 45 min

Serve: 6

Ingredients:

- Juice of ½ lemon
- 1 cup (240 ml) half-and-half
- ½ teaspoon guar or xanthan
- cups (0.9 L) chicken broth, divided
- 1 can (14 ounces, or 410 g) quartered artichoke hearts, drained
- 1 clove garlic, crushed
- stalks celery, finely chopped
- 1 small onion, finely chopped
- to 4 tablespoons (42 to 56 g) butter
- Salt or Vega-Sal
- Pepper

Instructions:

1. Melt the butter in a big skillet, then sauté the celery, onion, and garlic over low to medium heat. Shake from time to time.

2. Drain the hearts of the artichoke and pick off any rough leaf pieces left on.

3. Placed the heart of the artichoke in a food processor with the S-blade in place. Add 1/2 cup (120 ml) of chicken broth and guar gum and strain until a fine purée is made from the artichokes. In a saucepan, scrape the artichoke mixture, add the remaining chicken broth, and boil over medium-high heat.

4. Stir the onion and celery into the artichoke mixture until tender. Whisk on the half-and-half when it comes to a boil. Take it back to a boil, push in the juice of a lemon and stir again. To taste, apply salt and pepper. You can eat this right now, hot, or you can eat it cooled in summers.

Nutrition: 10 grams of carbohydrates and 3 grams of fiber each, with 7 grams of carbohydrates and 4 grams of protein, respectively.

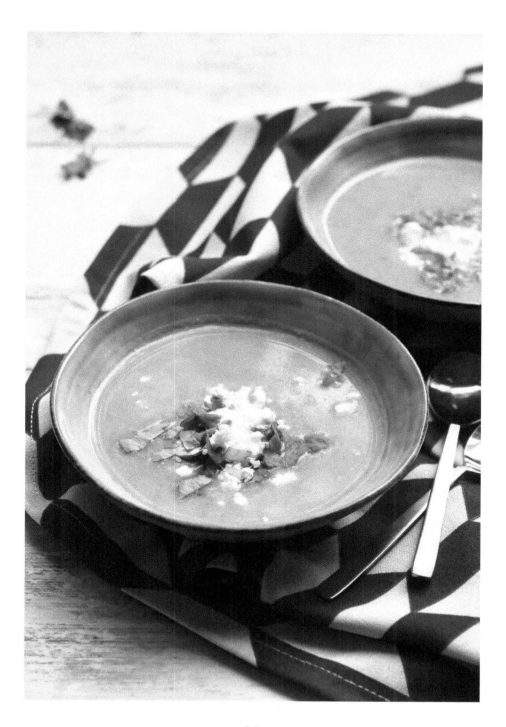

Curried Pumpkin Soup

Prep Time: 30 min

Cook Time: 30 min

Serve: 6

Ingredients:

- teaspoons curry powder
- ½ cup (120 ml) Carb Countdown dairy beverage
- 1½ cups (240 g) canned pumpkin
- 1 quart (960 ml) chicken broth
- 1 tablespoon (14 g) butter
- 1 clove garlic
- ¼ cup (40 g) minced onion
- Salt and pepper to taste

Instruction:

1. In a big saucepan, saute the garlic and onion in butter, heavy-bottomed saucepan with medium-low heat until only softened. Put in the broth of the chicken and cook for half an hour.

2. Mix in the dairy beverage Carb Countdown, canned pumpkin, and Curry Powder. Adjust to a boil and cook softly for a further 15 minutes.

3. To taste, incorporate salt and pepper, and then eat.

Nutrition: 6 servings, Each with 5 g protein; 7 g carbohydrate; 2 g dietary fiber; 5 g usable carbs.

Soap Aguacate

Prep Time: 30 min

Cook Time: 30 min

Serve: 4

Ingredients:

- ½ teaspoon salt or Vega-Sal
- tablespoons (8 g) chopped cilantro
- Canned green chilies or 1 or 2 canned jalapeños, if you like it hot!
- 2 scallions
- 1 ripe black avocado
- 1 quart (960 ml) chicken broth

Instructions:

1.Begin heating the broth. You can put it on the burner in a pan or put it in the microwave in a big microwaveable bowl.

2.Scrape the avocado out of its skin and into a food mixer with the S-blade in place as the broth is heating up.

3.Add the chilies, cilantro, scallions, and salt. Pulse all to cut together — you can add any bits of avocado or purée it flat, whatever you want.

4.Split the avocado mixture into 4 tiny soup bowls when the broth is hot. Spoon over the avocado mixture with the heated broth and eat.

Nutrition: 6 grams of carbohydrates and 3 grams of fiber, respectively, with 3 grams of available carbohydrates and 6 grams of protein.

Cheesy Onion Soup

Prep Time: 1 hour

Cook Time: 1 hour

Serve: 4

Ingredients:

- ½ cup (120 ml) Carb Countdown dairy beverage
- 1 medium onion
- 1 quart (960 ml) beef broth
- ½ cup (120 ml) heavy cream
- Guar or xanthan (optional)
- 1½ cups (180 g) shredded sharp cheddar cheese
- Salt and pepper to taste

Instructions:

1.In a large saucepan, add the beef broth and start heating it over a medium-high flame. Cut the paper-thin onion and apply it to the broth. Switch the heat down to low as the broth begins to boil and let the entire thing steam for 1 hour. You should do this ahead of time if you like; turn off the heat, let the entire thing cool, refrigerate it, and later do the rest. If you do this, before moving, lift the broth from heating again.

2.Stir in the cream and the dairy beverage Carb Timer softly. Now stir in the cheese, a little at a time, until all of it has melted in. If you want to thicken with guar or xanthan, stir with a ladle or spoon instead of a whisk, you don't want to sever the onion threads.

3.Garnish with salt and pepper and serve.

Nutrition: 24 g protein; 8 g carbohydrate; trace dietary fiber; 8 g usable carbs.

Cream of Potato Soup

Prep Time: 1 hour

Cook Time: 5 hours

Serve: 6

Ingredients:

- ½ cup (120 ml) Carb Countdown dairy beverage
- ½ cup (120 ml) heavy cream
- ½ cup (50 g) Ketones mix
- ½ cup (50 g) chopped onion
- ½ head cauliflower, chunked
- 1 quart (960 ml) chicken broth Guar or xanthan (optional)
- 5 scallions, sliced

Instructions:

1.in your slow cooker, put cauliflower, broth, and onion. Close and set the slow cooker to low and run for about 4 to 5 hours.

2.We used a hand mixer to purée the soup right in the slow cooker; so alternatively, you should pass the cauliflower and onion into your blender or food processor, along with 1 cup (240 ml) of broth. Purée until entirely smooth, and then blend into the Ketatoes, either way. If the cauliflower has been withdrawn from the slow cooker for purée, add the purée back in and whisk it back into the remaining broth.

3.Stir in the Carb Countdown and cream. If you believe it needs it, thicken it a little more with guar or xanthan.

4.To taste, apply salt and pepper and mix in the sliced scallions. Serve instantly hot or chill and serve as Vichyssoise.

Nutrition: 12 g protein, 13 g carbohydrate, 6 g dietary fiber, 7 g usable carbs.

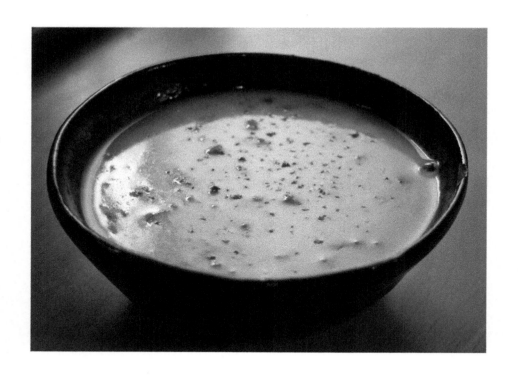

Swiss cheese and Broccoli Soup

Prep Time: 10 min

Cook Time: 1 hour

Serve: 6-8

Ingredients:

- Guar or xanthan
- cups (360 g) shredded Swiss cheese
- 1 cup (240 ml) heavy cream
- cup (500 ml) Carb Countdown dairy beverage
- 10 ounces (560 g) frozen chopped broccoli, thawed
- 28 ounces (400 ml) chicken broth
- tablespoon (28 g) butter
- tablespoons (420 g) minced onion

Instructions:

1.Sauté the onion into the butter in a big, heavy-bottomed saucepan until it is transparent. Put the broccoli and the chicken broth in the pan and cook for 20 to 30 minutes until the broccoli is very soft.

2.Mix in the Countdown Carb and some cream. Brought it to a simmer again.

3.Now mix in the cheese, a little at a time, allowing each batch to melt before adding any more. Thicken a bit with guar or xanthan when all the cheese is melted if you think it needs it, and then serve.

Nutrition: 20 g protein; 7 g carbohydrate; 2 g dietary fiber; 5 g usable carbs.

Tavern Soup

Prep Time: 8-10 hours

Cook Time: 1 hour

Serve: 8

Ingredients:

- 1/2 teaspoon hot pepper sauce
- 1 teaspoon salt or Vega-Sal
- 24 ounces (500 ml) light beer
- pound (900 g) sharp cheddar cheese, shredded
- 1 teaspoon pepper
- 1/2 cup (30.4 g) chopped fresh parsley
- 1/2 cup (60 g) shredded carrot
- 1/2 cup (60 g) finely diced green bell pepper
- 1/2 cup (60 g) finely diced celery
- Guar or xanthan
- quarts (3 L) chicken broth

Instructions:

1.Mix in your slow cooker celery, broth, green pepper, onion, parsley, and pepper. Close the slow cooker, set it to low, and let it steam for 6 to 8 hours (it won't hurt for a little longer).

2.To purée the vegetables in the slow cooker right there until the time is up, use a handheld blender to scoop them out with a slotted spoon, and purée them in the blender, and add them to the slow cooker.

3.Now swirl a little at a time in the cheese until it's all melted. Add the hot pepper sauce, beer, salt, or Vega-Sal, and mix until the foaming ends.

4.To thicken the broth, use guar or xanthan until it is about sour cream thickness. Cover the pot again, turn it too heavy, and simmer for an additional 20 minutes before eating.

Nutrition: 18 g protein, 3 g carbohydrate, trace dietary fiber, 3 g usable carbs.

Broccoli Blue Cheese Soup

Prep Time: 1 hour

Cook Time: 1 hour

Serve: 6-8

Ingredients:

- 1 cup (120 g) crumbled blue cheese
- ¼ cup (60 ml) heavy cream
- 1 pound (455 g) frozen broccoli, thawed
- 1½ quarts (1.4 L) chicken broth
- 1 cup (240 ml) Carb Countdown dairy beverage
- 1 turnip, peeled and diced
- tablespoons (28 g) butter
- cup (160 g) chopped onion

Instructions:

1.Sauté the onion in the butter over medium-low heat in a broad saucepan — you don't want it to tan.

2.Until the onion is soft and transpaarent, add the chicken broth and the turnip to your pot. Brought the blend to a boil and let it cook for 20 to 30 minutes over medium to low heat.

3.Put in the thawed broccoli and cook for the next 20 minutes.

4.With a slotted spon, scoop the vegetables out and put them in a Mixer. A ladleful broth is added to the mix, and the blender runs until the vegetables are finely puréed. Shift the mixture back to your pot. Stir in the Countdown Carbohydrate, the heavy cream, and the blue cheese. Simmer for the next 5 to 10 minutes stirring periodically, and serve.

Nutrition: 14 g protein; 9 g carbohydrate; 3 g dietary fiber; 6 g usable carbs.

Cream of Mushroom Soup

Prep Time: 6 hours

Cook Time: 1 1/2 hour

Serve: 5-7

Ingredients:

- ½ cup (120 g) light sour cream
- ½ cup (120 ml) heavy cream
- 1 quart (960 ml) chicken broth
- tablespoons (28 g) butter
- ¼ cup (25 g) chopped onion
- 8 ounces (225 g) mushrooms, sliced
- Guar or xanthan (optional)

Instruction:

1. Sauté the onion and mushrooms in the butter in a large, heavy skillet until the mushrooms soften and change color. Move them to a slow cooker. Put in the broth. Cover your slow cooker, set it low and let it cook for 5 to 6 hours.

2. Scrape out the vegetables with a slotted spoon when the time is up, and stick them in your blender or any food processor.

3. Add in enough broth to help them quickly process and finely purée them. Put the puréed vegetables back into the slow cooker, using a rubber scraper to clean out any last piece. Now whisk in

the heavy cream and sour cream and apply to taste the salt and pepper. If you think it deserves it, thicken the sauce a little with guar or xanthan. Serve asp.

Nutrition: 6 g protein, 5 g carbohydrate, 1 g dietary fiber, 4 usable carbs.

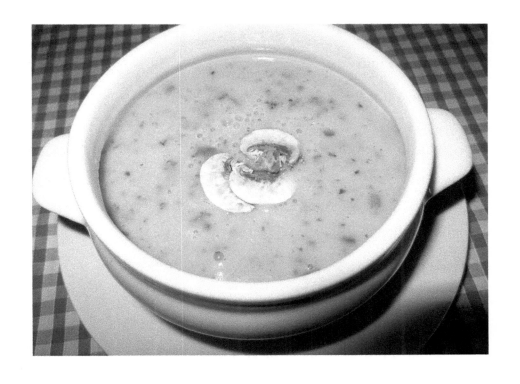

Olive Soup

Prep Time: 20 min

Cook Time: 1 hour

Serve: 6-8

Ingredients:

- Pepper
- Salt or Vega-Sal
- ¼ cup (60 ml) dry sherry
- ½ teaspoon guar or xanthan
- 1 cup (100 g) minced black olives (You can buy cans of minced black olives.)
- 1 cup (240 ml) heavy cream
- cups (0.9 L) chicken broth, divided

Instructions:

1. Put 1/2 cup (120 ml) of the chicken broth with the guar gum in the blender and pulse for a few moments. Pour the remainder of the stock and the olives into a saucepan and add the blended mixture.

2. Heat and then whisk in the milk before simmering. Return to a boil, stir in the sherry, then apply salt and pepper to taste.

Nutrition: 3,5 grams of carbohydrates and 1,1 g. of fiber, for a total of 2,5 grams of usable carbs and 2,5 grams of protein.

Salmon Soup

Prep time: 15 minutes

Cook time: 21 minutes

Serve: 4

Ingredients:

- 1 pound salmon fillets
- 1 tablespoon olive oil
- 1 cup carrots, peeled and chopped
- ½ cup celery stalk, chopped ¼ cup yellow onion, chopped 1 cup cauliflower, chopped 3 cups chicken broth
- Salt and ground black pepper, as required ¼ cup fresh parsley, chopped

Instructions:

1.Arrange a steamer trivet in the lower part of the Instant Pot and pour 1 cup of water.

2. Place the salmon fillets on top of trivet in a single layer.

3. Secure the lid and switch to the role of "Seal".

4. Cook on "Manual" with "High Pressure" for about 7-8 minutes.

5. Press "Cancel" and carefully do a "Quick" release.

6. Remove the lid and transfer the salmon onto a plate. Cut the salmon into bite sized pieces.

7. Remove the water and trivet from Instant Pot.

8. Add the oil in Instant Pot and select "Sauté". Then add the carrot, celery and onion and cook for about 5 minutes or until browned completely.

9. Press "Cancel" and stir in the cauliflower and broth.

10. Secure the lid and switch to the role of "Seal".

11. Cook on "Manual" with "High Pressure" for about 8 minutes.

12. Press "Cancel" and do a "Natural" release.

13. Remove the lid and stir in salmon pieces and black pepper until well combined.

14. Serve immediately with the garnishing of parsley.

Nutrition: Calories: 233 | fat: 11.6g | protein: 26.7g | carbs: 6g | net carbs: 4.2g | fiber: 1.8g

Cheesy Mushroom Soup

Prep Time: 15 minutes

Cook Time: 15 minutes

Serve: 4

Ingredients:

- 2 tablespoons olive oil
- 4 ounces fresh baby Portobello mushroom, sliced
- 4 ounces fresh white button mushrooms, sliced ½ cup yellow onion, chopped
- ½ teaspoon salt
- 1 teaspoon garlic, chopped
- 3 cups low-sodium vegetable broth
- 1 cup low-fat cheddar cheese

Instructions:

1.Heat the oil over normal heat in a medium saucepan and cook the mushrooms and onion with salt for approximately 5-7 minutes, stirring frequently.

2.Add the garlic, and sauté for about 1-2 minutes.

3.Stir in the broth and remove from the heat.

4.With a stick blender, blend the soup until mushrooms are chopped very finely.

5.In the pan, add the heavy cream and stir to combine.

6.Place the pan over medium heat and cook for about 3-5 minutes.

7.Remove from the heat.

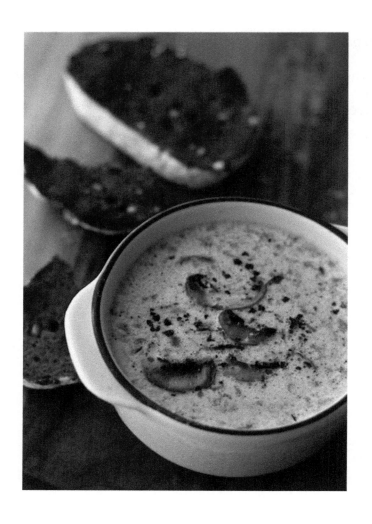

Herbed Lemon Chicken

Prep Time: 10 Minutes

Cook Time: 20-30 Minutes

Serve: 4 Serving

Ingredients:

- 2-3 T fresh chopped herbs (parsley, thyme, rosemary, chives, tarragon, etc.
- 1 T Dash of Desperation Seasoning
- Four teaspoons Luscious Lemon Oil (or oil, fresh lemon juice, and fresh lemon zest)
- 1 1/2 lbs. boneless, skinless chicken breasts (or thighs)

Instructions:

1.Preheat to medium-high heat (about 350) * outdoor grill *

2.In a large-pot, add all the ingredients and toss to cover.

3.Grill each side for 7-12 minutes until the beef is thoroughly cooked (check with the meat thermometer)

Char-Grilled Tuscan Chicken Kebabs

Ingredients:

- 3 T Apple Cider Vinegar
- 4 tbsp. Roasted Garlic Oil
- 2 T Tuscan Fantasy Seasoning
- 1 C Zucchini cut into ½ inch thick slices
- 1 C Cherry tomatoes*
- 1 C Green bell pepper cut-into 1" pieces
- 1 C Red bell-pepper cut into 1" pieces
- 1½ lb. Boneless chicken breasts cut into 1" pieces

Instructions:

1.Using a big zipper bag to add all the ingredients. Seal the bag and mix the marinade into the vegetables and poultry. Place in the refrigerator for up to one hour overnight. Preheat the outdoor grill to medium-high heat when ready to bake.

2.For best cooking results, thread meat and vegetables onto individual skewers, alternating them. Grill on either side for 5-7 minutes before you hit the target temperature. For better performance, use a meat thermometer.

Salmon at Home

Ingredients:

- 1 T Phoenix Sunrise Seasoning
- 1 lb. salmon filet with skin on

Instructions:

1.Preheat a nonstick pan for 1 minute on high flame.

2.Sprinkle seasoning over the salmon during the heating process (NOT on the skin side)

3.Decrease the heat to medium height.

4.Place the fish in the pan and let it cook for 4-6 minutes, seasoning side down depending on the thickness.

5.Lower the heat to medium-low.

6.Flip the fish down to the skin side and cook for 4-6 more minutes. (Less for medium / rare and well finished, more so.)

7.Withdraw from the sun and serve. Fish should slip to the plate right off the skin and on.

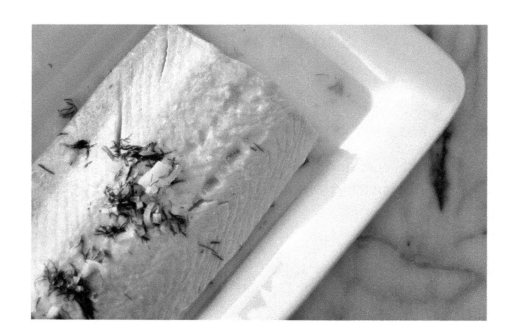

Simple Chicken Curry

Ingredients:

- Fresh cilantro for garnish if desired.
- 2 C fresh cauliflower, cut into 1" florets (NOT smaller- will overcook)
- 1/2 C water
- 1 tbsp. salt (optional)
- 1 T Garlic Gusto Seasoning
- 1 T Spices of India Seasoning
- 2 C diced tomatoes (fresh or canned)
- 1 C red bell pepper, seeded & chopped into 1" chunks
- 1.25 lbs. boneless-skinless-chicken thighs OR 1.5 lbs. boneless, skinless chicken breasts

Instructions:

1.Put a single layer of chicken on the bottom of a slow cooker.

2.Combine the pepper, onions, cloves, salt, and water in a shallow cup. Throw chicken over it.

3.Comb the chicken with cauliflower florets.

4.Cover and simmer for 6-8 hours, on low heat, until the chicken is fork-tender.

5.Ladle into four bowls and, if needed, garnish with cilantro.

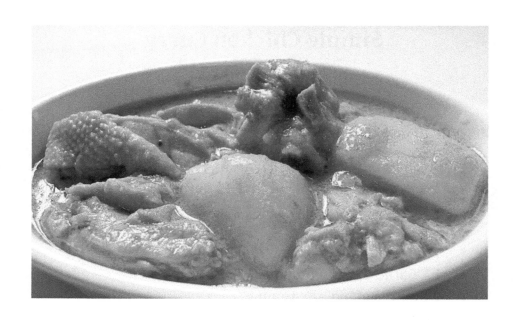

Juicy Stuffed

Ingredients:

- Nonstick cooking spray
- Four large portobello mushrooms, trimmed, stems removed.
- 8 T Cheese- blue, feta, or parmesan (optional)
- 1 T Garlic and Spring Onion Seasoning
- 4 T + 1T Italian Basil Infused Panko
- 1 large egg
- 1 1/4 lb. lean ground beef, chicken, or turkey (85-90% lean)

Instructions:

1.Preheat the oven to 350 ° C. Spray with nonstick cooking spray on a baking sheet.

2.Wash the stems from the mushrooms, cut, and extract them.

3.Take the roots and fine dice them.

4.Apply the stems and steak, bacon, 4 T panko, and Garlic & Spring Onion Seasoning to a large tub.

5.With your hands, combine the ingredients until well combined.

6.Divide the mixture of meat into four equal portions.

7.Pack the meat loosely into the mushroom caps.

8.For the leftover panko and cheese, spread uniformly.

9.Bake until completely baked for 25-30 minutes.

Stuffed Bruschetta Chicken

Ingredients:

- 4 T Italian Basil Infused Panko Breadcrumbs
- 4 tbsp. Roasted Garlic Oil
- 1 C bruschetta
- Four boneless skinless chicken breasts (about 1 1/2 lbs.)

Instructions:

1. Preheat the oven to 350 ° C.

2. To make a stuffing jar, slice chicken breasts.

3. Place the chicken breast with 1/4 C of bruschetta and place it in a baking dish.

4. Repeat the procedure for and breast of the chicken until they are all stuffed.

5. Drizzle the oil over each chicken breast similarly.

6. Sprinkle the panko with the chicken.

7. Bake for 23-33 minutes, until the chicken is cooked (180 degrees internal temp.)

8. Slicing and cooking!

Pork Tenderloins and Mushrooms

Prep Time: 10 minutes

Cook Time: 25 minutes

Serve: 4

Ingredients:

- on-stick cooking spray 1 Tablespoon garlic
- 1 Tablespoon marjoram
- 1 Tablespoon basil
- 1 Tablespoon onion
- 1 Tablespoon parsley
- 1 1/2 lbs. pork tenderloin (or beef tenderloin, or chicken breasts) 6 cups portobello mushroom caps, cut into chunks
- 1/2 C low sodium chicken broth
- 1 Tablespoon Stacey Hawkins Garlic Gusto or Garlic & Spring
- Onion Seasoning (or garlic, salt, black pepper, onion, paprika, and parsley)
- fresh parsley for garnish if desired

Instructions:

1.Spray a large skillet with cooking spray.

2.Preheat the stove to medium heat.

3.Place garlic and herbs into the skillet to cook with the cooking spray.

4.Allow the garlic and herbs to cook for 1 minute.

5.Place the pork tenderloin into the pan.

6.Generously season the pork tenderloin with the garlic gusto.

7.Sear the pork for 5 minutes and flip to the other side. Cook the other-side for another 1 minute.

8.Add the mushrooms, broth, and 2 tablespoons of water into the pan.

9.Cover the pan for 20 minutes.

10.Uncover and simmer for an additional 10,5 minutes till tender.

11.Garnish with marjoram. Serve hot.

Nutrition: Energy (calories): 737 kcal Protein: 30.32 g Fat: 62.95 g Carbohydrates: 14.39 g Calcium, Ca40 mg Magnesium, Mg48 mg Phosphorus, P443 mg

Garlic Shrimp & Broccoli

Prep Time: 15 min and 30 min marinade

Cook Time: 8 minutes

Serve: 4

Ingredients:

- 1/2 cup honey
- 1/4 cup soy sauce
- 1 teaspoon fresh grated ginger
- 2 tablespoons minced garlic
- 1/4 teaspoon red pepper flakes
- 1/2 teaspoon cornstarch
- 1-pound large shrimp, peeled, deveined, and tails removed if desired
- 2 tablespoon butter
- 2 cups chopped broccoli
- 1 teaspoon olive oil
- salt pepper

Instructions:

1.In a large-bowl, combine honey, soy sauce, ginger, garlic, red pepper flakes, and cornstarch. Add shrimp and toss to combine. Cover and refrigerate for 23 to 33 minutes.

2.Stir-fry in a cast iron pan:

3.In a big-nonstick skillet, heat 1 normal spoon of the butter and olive oil over medium-high heat. Cook and stir broccoli in the hot skillet until crisp-tender, occasionally stirring, 2 to 4 minutes. Remove broccoli from skillet.

4.Add shrimp mixture to hot skillet and stir-fry for 4-5 minutes or until shrimp are done. Stir in broccoli and add salt and pepper to taste.

5.Remove from the heat.

6.Serve with rice; your family will love it!

Nutrition: Energy (calories): 334 kcal Protein: 17.84 g Fat: 11.07 g Carbohydrates: 43.4 g Calcium, Ca100 mg Magnesium, Mg42 mg Phosphorus, P324 mg

Chicken with Garlic and Spring Onion Cream

Prep Time: 5 minutes

Cook Time: 15 minutes

Serve: 4

Ingredients:

- 6 medium chicken breasts
- 3 spoons butter or 3 espoons margarine 2 spoons all-purpose flour
- One-third cup chopped green onion Three-fourth cup chicken broth One-fourth teaspoon salt
- pepper
- 1 -2 tablespoon Dijon mustard (to taste) 1 cup plain yogurt

Instructions:

1.Heat a large skillet, add 1 tablespoon butter. Add chicken breasts to the pan. Cook for 10 minutes on medium heat, until browned on both sides. Remove and set aside on a plate.

2.Flour a chopping board and cut chicken breasts into thin strips when you're free from extra fat.

3.Melt 2 spoons butter in the same skillet. Stir in flour and cook for 2 minutes, stirring constantly. Gradually add chicken broth, mustard, salt, and pepper. (For a thicker sauce, add 2 tablespoons cornstarch dissolved in 1/2 cup cold water.)

4.Blend in yogurt. Add chicken strips and green onion. Cook until sauce bubbles and thickens, stirring occasionally.

5.Serve with plain white rice or boiled potatoes.

Nutrition: Energy (calories): 1172 kcal Protein: 132.83 g Fat: 63.49 g Carbohydrates: 9.7 g Calcium, Ca162 mg Magnesium, Mg155 mg Phosphorus, P1073 mg

Pan-Seared Beef Tips and Mushrooms

Prep Time: 10 minutes

Cook Time: 25 minutes

Serve: 4

Ingredients:

- 1 1/2 lbs. lean beef cut into 1 chunk (London broil, filet, strip steak, etc.)
- 1/2 T salt 1/2 T pepper 1/2 T garlic
- nonstick cooking spray
- 4 C mushrooms (either small, whole mushrooms or larger ones cut into quarters)
- 1 C low sodium beef broth 11/2 teaspoons fresh garlic 11/2 teaspoons parsley 11/2 teaspoons onion

Instructions:

1.Sprinkle beef with salt, pepper, and garlic.

2.Coat large skillet with nonstick cooking spray. Heat over medium-high heat and add beef. Cook about 8-10 minutes, stirring frequently or until beef is browned on all sides and no pink remains.

3.Add mushrooms to the skillet. Pour beef broth and boil. Cover and cook over low-heat for 15 minutes.

4.While beef simmers in mushroom sauce, combine garlic, parsley, and onion in a food processor fitted with a steel blade. Pulse a few times until minced.

5.Add garlic mixture to beef and mushrooms and simmer covered for 10 minutes more.

6.Place in the serving bowl and season with parsley. As an alternative, if desired, top with gouda cheese.

Nutrition: Energy (calories): 379 kcal Protein: 42.49 g Fat: 12.44 g Carbohydrates: 25.55 g Calcium, Ca66 mg Magnesium, Mg69 mg

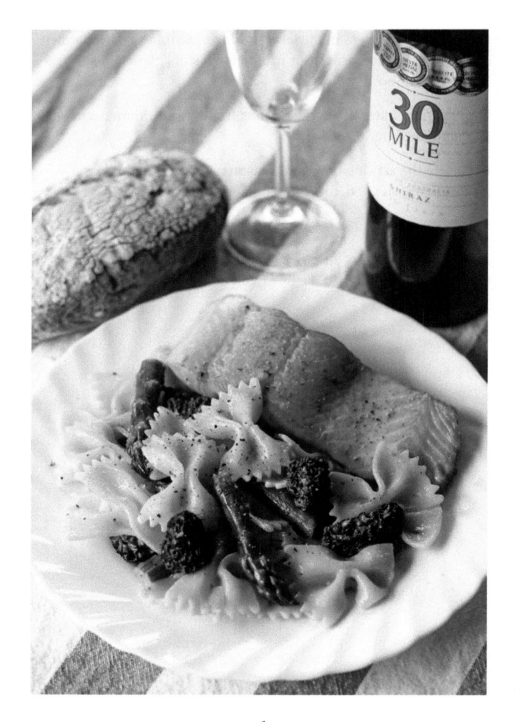

Creamy Skillet Chicken and Asparagus

Prep Time: 5 minutes

Cook Time: 20 minutes

Serve: 4

Ingredients:

- 1 1/2 tablespoon extra-virgin olive oil
- Salt and fresh-ground pepper to taste, 4 (1 pound) boneless skinless chicken breasts
- 2 spoons Italian Seasoning 1 tablespoon butter
- 1-pound asparagus stalks trimmed and cut into thirds 1 yellow onion sliced
- 1 cup fat-free half & half 1/2 tablespoon all-purpose 1/3 cup grated Parmesan flour
- Lemon slices of salt and fresh ground pepper to taste for garnishing chopped parsley for garnishing freshly rubbed parmesan to garnish

Instructions:

1.Heat a big nonstick omelet pan over medium-high heat. Add olive oil and swirl. Season chicken with salt and pepper and Italian season. Add chicken to the pan and sauté until the tops are brown, about 4 minutes, then flip and cook another 4,3-5,3 minutes, or until golden.

2.Remove chicken from pan and keep warm. Add butter to the pan, asparagus, onion, and sauté until the asparagus is tender, about 4 mins.

3.Season the asparagus. Sprinkle in the flour, constantly stirring, until the mixture is homogenized and bubbly. Gradually add the 1/2 cup of half and half, constantly stirring, then add parmesan cheese, garlic, lemon juice, salt, and pepper.

4.Cook until sauce thickens, about 2 minutes. Taste and adjust seasoning. Stir in the rest of the half and half. Add chicken back into the pan to reheat and toss together with the sauce.

5.Remove from heat and onto the plates. Serve and garnish with lemon-slices, parsley, and parmesan.

Nutrition: Energy (calories): 703 kcal Protein: 110.07 g Fat: 18.54 g Carbohydrates: 19.52 g Calcium, Ca190 mg Magnesium, Mg171 mg

Seared with Lemon-Basil Butter

Prep Time: 10 minutes

Cook Time: 20 minutes

Serve: 4-6

Ingredients:

- 3 tablespoons unsalted butter
- 1 and one-half teaspoons fresh lemon juice 1 large garlic clove, finely chopped
- One-fourth teaspoon salt, plus additional for seasoning
- One-fourth teaspoon fresh ground black pepper, plus additional for seasoning
- 1 and one-half tablespoons basil leaves, chopped fresh 3 tablespoons olive oil
- 3 mahi-mahi fillet

Instructions:

1.Melt the butter in a small-saucepan over low flame. Add garlic, lemon juice, salt, pepper, and basil. Cook over low heat for 1 minute, regularly stirring the mixture so the butter doesn't burn. Turn off the flame and remove the prepared sauce from the heat. Using a wooden spoon, place the sauce in a bowl, preferably stainless steel, and cool it to room temperature for an even better result. Give it a whisk just before you are ready to use it.

2.Preheat an oven to 450°F. Place a grill-pan over medium flame and add 2 tablespoons olive oil.

3.Season the mahi-mahi fillets with salt and pepper and drizzle 1/4 of the lemon-basil sauce over them. Reserve the remaining sauce for later use.

4.Sear the Mahi mahi on both sides for approximately 2-3 minutes until the fish is opaque and cooked through. Remove the fish-fillet from the grill pan and place them on a baking sheet coated with baking paper.

5.Add the remaaining olive oil to the grill pan you used to cook the fish. Add the fillet to the grill pan and finish cooking the mahi-mahi, searing the top for an additional 1-2 minutes.

6.Serve with any side dish you choose. Eating the fish with a fresh green salad drizzled with lemon-basil sauce is a great combination.

Nutrition: Energy (calories): 222 kcal Protein: 10.19 g Fat: 18.28 g Carbohydrates: 4.76 g Calcium, Ca46 mg Magnesium, Mg12 mg Phosphorus, P198 mg

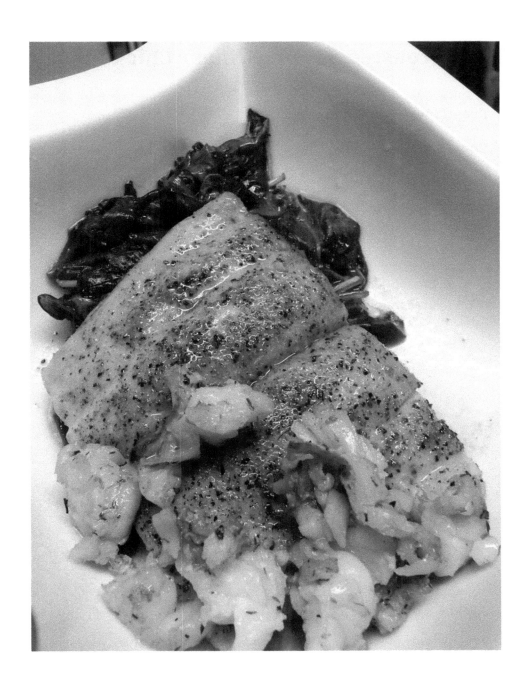

Toasted Sesame Ginger Chicken

Prep Time: 10 minutes

Cook Time: 15 minutes

Serve: 4

Ingredients:

- 4 teaspoons olive oil
- 4 teaspoons orange zest
- 1 1/2 lbs. boneless-skinless-chicken breast 1 Tablespoon toasted sesame seeds
- 1 Tablespoon garlic
- 1 Tablespoon onion powder 1 Tablespoon red pepper
- 1 Tablespoon ground ginger 1 Tablespoon salt
- 1 Tablespoon pepper
- 1 Tablespoon lemon

Instructions:

1.Remove the small fillet from each chicken breast, and cut and reserve.

2.Preheat oven to 375 degrees F.

3.Cook sesame seeds over medium heat in oil until they are crisp and turn a little brown.

4.Add chicken and cook for 5,3 minutes on each side, or until it is slightly crispy.

5.Place the chicken-onions, and garlic in a baking dish, and sprinkle with the seasonings. Bake for another 15 minutes, stirring occasionally.

6.Meanwhile, stir together teriyaki sauce and cornstarch in a small saucepan.

7.Bring to a boil, and cook for 1 minute without stirring.

8.Remove the chicken and serve with the glaze.

Nutrition: Energy (calories): 369 kcal Protein: 16.84 g Fat: 15.27 g Carbohydrates: 41.12 g Calcium, Ca58 mg Magnesium, Mg50 mg Phosphorus, P185 mg

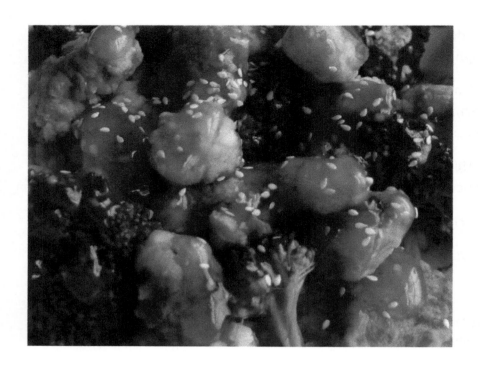

Tender and Tasty Fish Tacos

Prep Time: 10 minutes

Cook Time: 15 minutes

Serve: 4

Ingredients:

- 1 3/4 lbs. cod or haddock (wild-caught)
- 1 capful (1 Tablespoon) Phoenix Sunrise Seasoning or cumin, cilantro, garlic, onion, red pepper, paprika, parsley, salt & pepper (or low sodium taco seasoning)
- 4 little spoons Stacey Hawkins Roasted Garlic Oil or oil of your choice and fresh garlic
- your favorite taco condiments

Instructions:

1.Thaw fish in a separate bowl from other ingredients and heat frying pan at medium (350º - 375º F)

2.Preheat oven at 400º F

3.Line a baking sheet with parchment paper

4.Cut fish into cubes evenly about 1/2"x1/2". Prepare the oil mixture with the chopping knife by adding the Stacey Hawkins Roasted Garlic Oil or Olive Oil to the oiling bowl and fresh garlic cloves with the skins still on. Extra garlic makes food taste good.

5.Preheat a clean frying pan on medium to high heat

6.Add fish to the frying pan and allow it to cook for 2-4 minutes, or until it becomes opaque. With your cooking tweezers or fork, flip the fish to cook the other side for an additional 2-4 minutes. Keep fish-warm in the oven while preparing tortillas.

7.To prepare the tortillas, heat the frying pan at medium heat, add tortilla to the pan, and heat on each side for 20 seconds (you might need to add a small amount of oil). To keep the tortillas warm, put the tortillas in the oven at 400º F and close the door.

8.Remove tortillas from the oven and immediately add fish and other ingredients and fold it all together.

Nutrition: Energy (calories): 202 kcal Protein: 32.59 g Fat: 6.08 g Carbohydrates: 2.02 g Calcium, Ca25 mg Magnesium, Mg44 mg Phosphorus, P458 mg

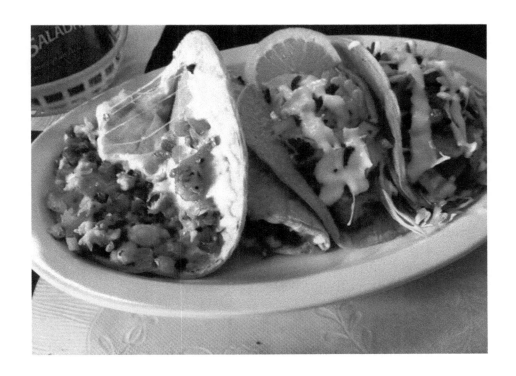

Sausage Stuffed Mushrooms

Prep Time: 5 minutes

Cook Time: 25 minutes

Serve: 4

Ingredients:

- 4 large portobello mushrooms (caps and stems) 1 1/2 pounds lean Italian sausage (85-94% lean) 1 capful (1 Tablespoon) chopped garlic
- 1 capful (1 Tablespoon) chopped chives
- 1 capful (1 Tablespoon) garlic powder
- 1 capful (1 Tablespoon) onion powder
- 1 capful (1 Tablespoon) salt and pepper to taste

Instructions:

1.Preheat the oven to 425 degrees F.

2.Sauté the sausage with the garlic and onion/garlic powders in a skillet without coloring it. Place the mushroom caps on a plate.

3.Mix the salt and pepper with the bread crumbs and stuff it inside the mushroom caps. Stuff the sausage mixture in the mushroom caps.

4.Spoon about a teaspoon of oil over the cap and place it stem side up on a cookie sheet.

5.Bake the caps for about 23 minutes or until the stuffing is fully cooked. Garnish with chives.

Nutrition: Energy (calories): 645 kcal Protein: 29.16 g Fat: 54.06 g Carbohydrates: 11.38 g Calcium, Ca49 mg Magnesium, Mg47 mg Phosphorus, P429 mg

Smoky Chipotle Shrimp and Tomatoes

Ingredients:

- 2 T fresh cilantro, chopped (optional)
- 1/2 large lime, juiced (optional)
- 1 T (one capful) Cinnamon Chipotle Seasoning
- 1 C diced tomatoes (unflavored, no sugar added)
- 1 1/2 lbs. wild-caught shrimp, shelled, deveined, and tails removed
- 1 C scallions (whites and greens) or chopped onion
- 4 tbsp. Roasted Garlic Oil

Instructions:

1.Heat oil over medium-high-heat in a medium-sized frying pan.

2.Put the onion and cook until translucent, for 2 minutes. Add shrimp and cook on each-side for 1 minute. Connect the chipotle tomatoes and cinnamon seasoning.

3.Cook for an extra 2-3 minutes until the tomatoes and shrimp are heated and opaque.

4.Drizzle and substitute the cilantro with the lemon juice. Serve it hot.

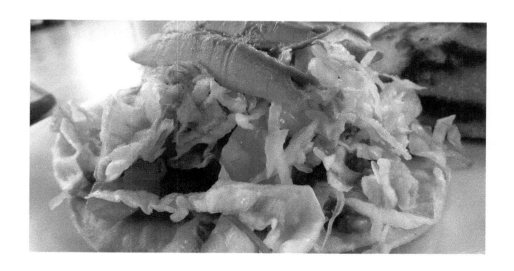

Simply Scrumptious Bruschetta

Ingredients:

- 4 tbsp. Balsamic Mosto Cot to
- 1 T Garlic Gusto Seasoning
- 1 tbsp. Viva Italian Blend
- 2 C fresh tomatoes, diced (you can use unseasoned, no sugar added canned tomatoes as well)

Instructions:

1.Place all the ingredients in a small-bowl and cover them with a toss.

2.Let it rest for 20 minutes, and then enjoy it.

3.It can be placed in an airtight-container and kept refrigerated for one week.

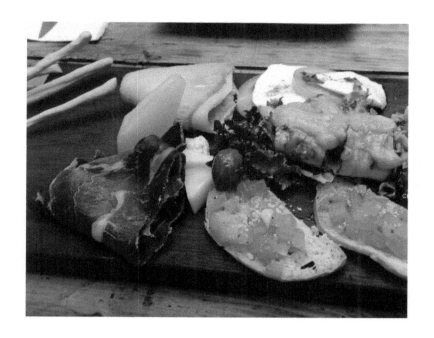

Rosemary Pulled Pork

Ingredients:

- 1 tbsp. Dash of Desperation Seasoning
- 1 1/2 T Rosemary Versatility Seasoning
- 1 C water
- 3 lbs. pork loin, excess fat removed

Instructions:

1.Place all the ingredients in order in the crockpot. Place the lid on and let it cook on low for 8-10 hours. The average size of the meat can depend on timing and tenderness.

2.It will take a little less time for smaller, longer parts, and it will take a little longer for narrower, stockier cuts (or those with bones).

3.Remove the lid when ready, and remove any bones carefully. Shred the meat using two big forks and throw it to cover in the juices in the crockpot.

4.Serve warm over salads or cauliflower rice as an entree. Superbly chilled over vegetables or on zero carb rolls as a sandwich.

Zesty Chicken with Artichokes and Garlic

Ingredients:

- 1/4 C green onions (scalions) tops only for garnish 1 T Skinny Scampi Seasoning 1 T Garlic Gusto Seasoning
- One 12-15oz. jar artichoke-hearts IN WATER NOT OIL drained well & chopped.
- 1½ lb. boneless-chicken-breasts, cut into 1" cubes 4 tbsp. Roasted Garlic Oil

Instructions:

1.Heat the Roasted-Garlic Oil in a pan in a large skillet over medium-high heat.

2.Include the chicken and cook on either side for 5-7 minutes, until the chicken is painted and solid.

3.Attach seasonings and artichokes. Turn the heat-to-low and simmer until the artichokes are sufficiently heated, and the chicken is completely cooked for an additional 5 minutes.

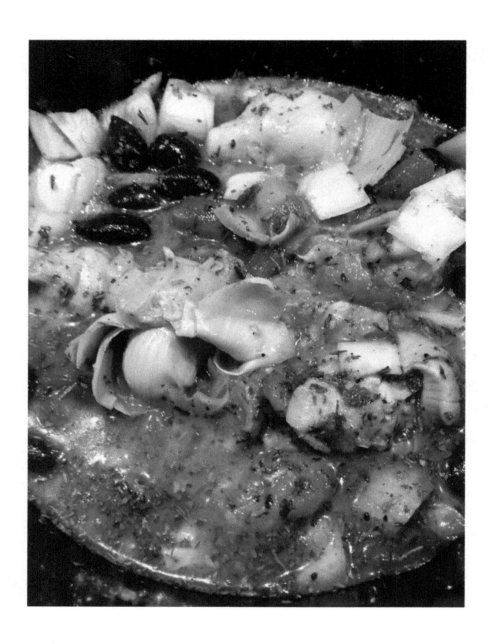

Crispy Baked Scampi Chicken

Ingredients:

- 4 T Lemon Pepper Infused Panko Bread Crumbs
- 1 T Skinny Scampi Seasoning
- 2 lbs. boneless, skinless chicken thighs, all visible fat removed

Instructions:

1.Preheat the oven to 350 ° C.

2.Place the chicken in one layer of a roasting oven.

3.Using Skinny Scampi Seasoning to sprinkle chicken.

4.Sprinkle the Lemon Pepper Panko with the chicken.

5.Bake until thoroughly fried, 30-40 minutes.

6.Take out froom the oven, leave to rest for about 5,3 minutes, and serve.

No Carb Garlic "Rolls"

Ingredients:

- 1 T Garlic & Spring Onion Seasoning
- 1 T cream cheese
- 1 T grated Parmesan cheese
- 1/8 tbsp. cream of tartar
- Three large eggs, separated

Instructions:

1.Preheat the oven to 300 ° F.

2.Separate the white and egg yolks into two wide cups.

3.Apply the tartar cream to a cup with the whites. Beat on high, using an electric-mixer, until very rigid peaks develop. And put aside.

4.Apply the remaining ingredients and the yolks to the dish. Beat together on high, using an electric mixer until all ingredients are combined.

5.Pour over the whites of the egg yolks and fold them softly until fully mixed.

6.Line 2 cookie sheets OR GENEROUSLY brush with nonstick cooking spray or silicone baking mats. Use a large spoon to put a dollop of egg mixture on the mat and spread it on a scale. DO NOT make them too thin, or they're going to roast and crisp. For better results, keep the egg mixture about 1/3 "deep. "Repeat the process to produce 12" rolls.

7.Take out from the oven and bake for 30 minutes. While still mildly warm, extract from your oven and place to cool aside.

8.The bread will be crispy in texture as it comes right out of the oven.

9.Place it in a zipper-type bag until cooled, and it will turn into fluffy, pliable bread that is delicious overnight!

Pan-Seared Lemon Tarragon Cod

Prep Time: 5 Minutes

Cook Time: 15 Minutes

Serve: 4 Serving

Ingredients:

- 1 3/4 lbs. cod fillets- fresh or frozen and thawed
- 4 tbsp. Luscious Lemon Oil
- 1 Tablespoon Rockin' Ranch Seasoning (or garlic, lemon, tarragon, pepper, onion, salt, and pepper)

Instructions:

1.Using a large frying pan to add oil, and cook over medium-high heat. Cut cod into 2″ chunks while the oil is heating.

2.Heat oil over medium-high-heat in a wide frying pan.

3.Break the cod into 2" chunks when boiling the oil.

4.Add fish to the pan while the oil is hot and cook on either side for 2-3 minutes, browning slightly. To be fully cooked and ready to eat, fish can take between 6-8 minutes.

5.It's done until the fish is translucent and flaky. Serve instantly.

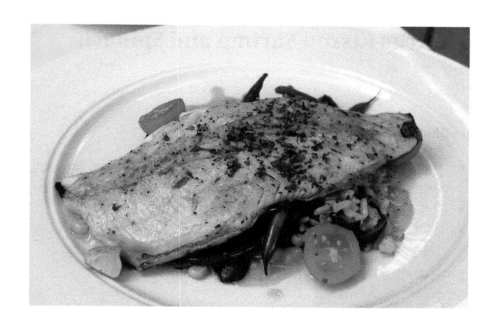

Citrus Kissed Shrimp and Spinach

Ingredients:

- 6 cups baby spinach greens, arugula greens, beet greens, or a combination
- 2 T Simply Brilliant Seasoning
- 1 1/2 lbs. wild-caught, raw shrimp, cleaned and tails removed
- 4 tbsp. Luscious Lemon Oil

Instructions:

1.Heat oil over medium-high-heat in a wide frying pan. Sprinkle with seasoning and put shrimp. Stir to cover and cook for about 3-4 minutes.

2.Switch the shrimp over once using tongs and cook for one minute. To the pan, add the vegetables. Toss it to coat it. Let the greens cook until wilted, for 1-2 minutes. Serve it warm.

Zesty Turkey and Kale Chili

Ingredients:

- 2 C chopped vegetables* (eggplant, zucchini, mushroom, etc.)
- 2 C chopped kale
- 2 T Zesty White Chili Seasoning
- 1 lb. ground turkey
- 2 C diced tomatoes
- 4 tbsp. Roasted Garlic Oil

Instructions:

1. In a medium-sized kettle, apply oil and fire over low heat.

2. Sprinkle with seasoning and substitute ground turkey.

3. Cook, stirring regularly, for 4,3-5,3 minutes, until the turkey is opaque.

4. Add the remaining ingredients, blend well, and reduce heat to mild.

5. Cover the pot and cook for 10,5 minutes, until the vegetables are tender.

6. Offer over some cauliflower rice.

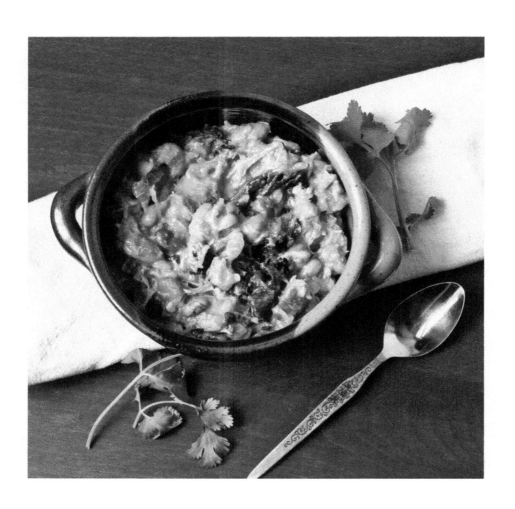

Muscle Meatballs

Prep Time: 15 minutes

Cook Time: 20 minutes

Serve: 3

Ingredients:

- 1 1/2 lb. extra-lean ground turkey breast 2 egg whites
- 1/2 cup of toasted wheat-germ 1/4 cup fast-cooking oats
- 1 tbsp. of whole linseed seeds
- 1 tbsp. of grated parmesan cheese One-half tsp. All-purpose seasoning 1/4 tsp. ground black pepper

Instructions:

1.Preheat the furnace to 400° F. Use cooking spray to cover a large baking dish.

2.In a container, mix all the ingredients.

3.Make and place 16 meatballs in the baking dish.

4.Bake the meatballs for 7 minutes and turn them around. Bake for 8–13 minutes longer, or until the center is no longer pink.

Nutrition: Energy (calories): 460 kcal Protein: 77.65 g Fat: 9.13 g Carbohydrates: 16.9 g Calcium, Ca78 mg Magnesium, Mg151 mg

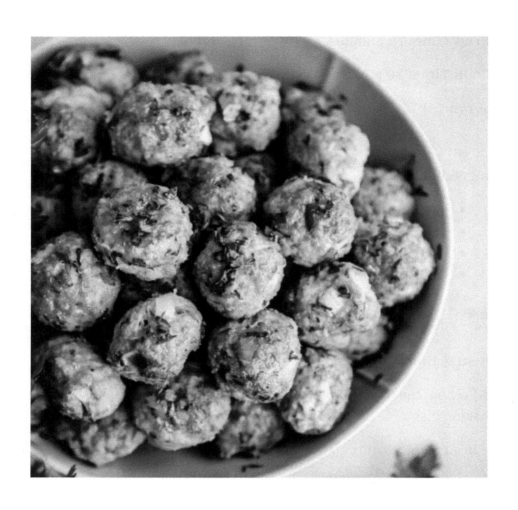

Lightning Source UK Ltd.
Milton Keynes UK
UKHW020652120521
383581UK00005B/30